REVOLUTIONIZING

DIABETES

MANAGEMENT

Innovative Therapies for Better
Health

Uncover The Latest
Breakthroughs In Diabetes
Therapy And Regain Control
Of Your Life

DR. BRIDGET PROMISE

Table of Contents

CHAPTER ONE

Introduction

Diabetes is a chronic metabolic illness that has emerged as a major worldwide health problem. With its growing prevalence, proper management and treatment options are essential.

Diabetes treatment has developed throughout time, with a shift from conventional techniques to new, patient-centered approaches.

This journey represents not just medical scientific improvements, but also the rising need for more individualized and accessible healthcare. In this discussion, we will look at the principles of diabetes, the historical development of its management, the current issues in diabetes care, and the potential landscape of emerging approaches to diabetes therapy.

Understanding Diabetes

Diabetes mellitus, sometimes known as diabetes, is a collection of metabolic illnesses characterized by persistently increased blood sugar levels.

This disease is caused by the body's inability to create enough insulin, poor insulin usage, or a combination of the two. Insulin, a hormone generated by the pancreas, plays an important function in blood sugar regulation by enabling glucose absorption into cells for energy.

Diabetes is classified into two types: type 1 and type 2. Type 1 diabetes is an autoimmune disease in which the immune system assaults and kills the pancreas' insulin-producing beta cells. Individuals with Type 1 diabetes need insulin treatment for the rest of their lives.

Type 2 diabetes, on the other hand, is defined by insulin resistance, which occurs when the body's cells do not react properly to insulin. This kind is often related to lifestyle problems such as poor nutrition, inactivity, and obesity. While Type 1 diabetes is often diagnosed in childhood or adolescence, Type 2 diabetes may develop at any age, and is frequently diagnosed later in life.

Diabetes has ramifications that go beyond high blood sugar levels. It may cause a variety of issues that affect the heart, kidneys, eyes, and nerves. Effective diabetes management is critical for preventing or delaying these consequences and improving the quality of life for diabetics.

Diabetes Management's Evolution

Significant advancements in diabetes care have occurred throughout history, showing the constant quest for viable therapies.

Sir Frederick Banting and Charles Best's discovery of insulin in the early twentieth century transformed diabetic therapy. Insulin treatment has become a life-saving medicine for people with Type 1 diabetes, enabling them to live more normal lives.

As our knowledge of diabetes grew, so did the number of medications available. Oral drugs including metformin, sulfonylureas, and thiazolidinediones have emerged as viable treatments for Type 2 diabetes. Continuous glucose monitoring (CGM) and insulin pumps were technical advances that allowed for more accurate regulation of blood sugar levels. These improvements enabled people with diabetes to actively engage in their care and make educated treatment choices.

CHAPTER TWO

Diabetes Care's Current Obstacles

Despite advances in diabetes treatment, several problems remain, impeding optimum care and results.

One of the most pressing issues is the growing worldwide incidence of diabetes, which is being exacerbated by lifestyle changes, urbanization, and an aging population.

Access to healthcare, especially in low-income areas, remains a key problem, in preventing diabetes from being diagnosed and managed on time.

Another issue is sticking to treatment programs. Diabetes management requires a complex strategy that includes medication, lifestyle changes, and frequent monitoring. However, financial level, cultural views, and psychological well-being may all have an impact on an individual's capacity to follow these suggestions.

Healthcare inequities worsen these issues, emphasizing the need for more inclusive and patient-centered methods.

Diabetes complications, such as cardiovascular disease, renal failure, and eye difficulties, continue to be major concerns. The importance of early discovery and action in preventing or mitigating these consequences cannot be overstated. Furthermore, the economic impact of diabetes, which includes both direct medical expenditures and indirect costs such as lost productivity, offers a significant challenge to healthcare systems globally.

Innovative Diabetes Treatment Methods

With the introduction of novel techniques that promote tailored care, technology integration, and holistic well-being, the diabetes treatment landscape is undergoing a paradigm change. Personalized medicine is gaining popularity, informed by genetic and biomarker data. The possibility of more effective and focused therapies lies in tailoring treatment programs based on an individual's unique genetic composition and reaction to drugs.

Technological advancements have resulted in the development of wearable gadgets and smartphone apps that allow people to monitor and control their diabetes in real-time. Continuous glucose monitoring (CGM) devices, when combined with insulin pumps, provide for more accurate regulation of blood sugar levels, lowering the risk of hypo- and hyperglycemia. These technologies not only improve medication effectiveness but also encourage a more proactive and involved approach to diabetes management.

Telemedicine has emerged as an important technique in diabetes treatment, especially in terms of enhancing access to healthcare services. Remote monitoring, virtual consultations, and digital platforms for teaching and support all help to make healthcare more patient-centric and accessible. Telemedicine overcomes geographical boundaries by enabling people to interact with healthcare professionals and get timely advice.

Furthermore, research into innovative therapeutic techniques, such as gene therapy and regenerative medicine, shows promise for diabetes treatment in the future.

These novel approaches seek to target the underlying causes of diabetes, with the possibility for disease transformation rather than symptom control.

Finally, since the discovery of insulin, diabetes care has progressed from a one-size-fits-all strategy to a more individualized and technologically driven paradigm. Despite existing hurdles, continued diabetes research and innovation have the potential to alter the lives of millions of people impacted by this chronic illness.

The future of diabetes care is bright, opening the way for better outcomes and a greater quality of life for persons living with diabetes by adopting tailored treatment programs, utilizing technology breakthroughs, and tackling healthcare inequities.

Personalized Medicine In Diabetes Management

With the advent of customized medicine, the landscape of diabetes care has experienced a revolutionary transformation in recent years.

This method tailors medical therapy to the unique qualities of each patient, understanding that in the world of healthcare, one size does not fit all. In the context of diabetes, customized medicine has considerably improved treatment accuracy and efficacy, allowing patients to get more focused and efficient care.

Technological Progress In Glucose Monitoring

Continuous glucose monitoring (CGM) is a critical component of individualized diabetes therapy. Traditional blood glucose monitoring techniques, such as fingerstick blood glucose testing, only provide intermittent snapshots of blood sugar levels. CGM devices, on the other hand, give real-time data, providing a full picture of glucose changes throughout the day. This technology not only helps patients to make better-informed decisions about their food choices and insulin doses, but it also allows healthcare practitioners to more precisely adjust treatment programs.

Modern CGM systems have features like as alarms for high or low blood sugar readings, giving patients and healthcare providers timely notifications.

This preventive strategy aids in the prevention of extreme swings and lowers the risk of diabetes-related problems. Furthermore, CGM device data may be readily shared with healthcare practitioners, supporting a collaborative and educated approach to diabetes treatment.

CHAPTER THREE

Insulin Delivery Systems Are Being Revolutionized

Insulin, a crucial hormone for blood sugar regulation, has witnessed considerable developments in delivery technologies.

Traditional insulin injections, although effective, may be uncomfortable and contribute to poor adherence to treatment programs. Insulin pumps and smart pens have transformed insulin delivery, offering more precise control and improving the overall quality of life for those with diabetes.

Insulin pumps continuously provide insulin throughout the day, simulating the normal insulin release of a healthy pancreas. They also allow for bolus dosages throughout meals, giving you more options for controlling post-meal glucose increases. In contrast, smart insulin pens provide a portable and user-friendly alternative to regular injections. Some versions also work with smartphone applications to manage insulin dosages, check glucose levels, and get individualized suggestions.

These advances not only make insulin delivery easier but also improve glycemic control, lowering the risk of hyperglycemia and hypoglycemia. As a consequence, people with diabetes may live more flexible and active lives.

Diabetes Control Nutritional Strategies

Nutrition is crucial in diabetes care, and customized medicine has an impact on dietary recommendations. Individuals with diabetes may now benefit from tailored nutritional strategies that take into account their specific metabolic profiles, lifestyle, and tastes, rather than following general dietary recommendations.

Genetic testing, for example, may disclose how a person metabolizes various nutrients, allowing dietary programs to be tailored to optimal blood sugar management. Furthermore, advances in nutritional research have resulted in the creation of specific diets, such as low-carbohydrate or Mediterranean diets, which have shown promising outcomes in the management of diabetes.

Furthermore, tailored nutrition entails more than just limiting particular meals; it also includes time and quantity management. Individuals may change their food choices based on real-time data, maximizing their nutritional intake to maintain stable blood sugar levels, when integrated with glucose monitoring equipment.

The Special Effects Of Substantial Activities On Blood Sugar

Regular physical exercise is essential for diabetes control, and individualized techniques take an individual's fitness level, preferences, and general health state into consideration. Individualizing exercise routines improves adherence and increases the advantages of physical activity in blood sugar management.

Technology also plays an important role in this regard. Wearable fitness trackers and smartwatches not only measure activity levels but may also reveal how various kinds and intensities of exercise influence blood sugar levels. This knowledge enables people to make educated decisions regarding their physical exercise routines, maximizing the beneficial influence on their diabetes control.

CHAPTER FOUR
The Psychosocial Aspects Of Diabetes

The psychological elements of diabetes are sometimes overlooked, although they are critical to providing comprehensive and customized treatment.

Diabetes treatment includes recognizing and managing patients' emotional and psychological well-being in addition to medicines, insulin levels, and food choices.

The relevance of mental health in diabetes care is recognized by personalized medicine. Psychosocial assistance, such as counseling and education, is an important component of tailored care programs. Addressing stress, anxiety, and depression, which may influence both physical and mental health, is critical for attaining optimum diabetes management results.

Furthermore, support groups and online forums allow people with diabetes to share their experiences, struggles, and accomplishments. These communities provide a sense of belonging and understanding, which alleviates feelings of loneliness and promotes general well-being.

Finally, customized medicine has transformed diabetes care in many ways, from the accuracy of medicinal treatments to the use of technology in monitoring and lifestyle control. Healthcare practitioners may provide more effective and individualized diabetes management measures by identifying and treating the particular peculiarities of each patient's situation, eventually increasing the quality of life for people living with this chronic illness.

Emerging Pharmaceuticals And Treatment Protocols

The diabetes management landscape is always changing due to the introduction of new drugs and treatment strategies. These developments are critical in improving patient outcomes, increasing glycemic control, and lowering the risk of diabetic complications.

Researchers and pharmaceutical firms have spent years researching novel treatment methods to address the complicated nature of diabetes.

One major advancement in diabetes medicine is the introduction of SGLT-2 inhibitors and GLP-1 receptor agonists. SGLT-2 inhibitors, such as empagliflozin and canagliflozin, function by preventing glucose reabsorption in the kidneys and boosting its excretion via urine. This technique lowers blood glucose levels and has been found to have considerable cardiovascular advantages, making them an important addition to the therapy arsenal.

Similarly, GLP-1 receptor agonists such as liraglutide and dulaglutide imitate the effect of incretin hormones by increasing insulin production while suppressing glucagon release. These drugs not only help with glucose management but also help with weight reduction, making them especially beneficial for those with type 2 diabetes who are obese.

Furthermore, novel insulin formulations aiming at enhancing convenience and effectiveness have been developed in the field. Insulins with ultra-rapid onset and duration, such as lispro and aspart, provide more flexibility in insulin dosage around meals. Long-acting insulins, such as degludec and glargine U300, offer longer durations of action, allowing for a once-daily dose and improved blood glucose stability.

Alternative And Complementary Therapies

Complementary and alternative treatments are gaining acceptance as adjuncts to conventional diabetes therapy, in addition to established pharmaceutical approaches. Integrating these treatments into a holistic treatment plan may provide diabetic patients with extra tools to enhance their overall health.

Mind-body techniques like yoga and meditation have shown potential in terms of stress reduction and glycemic management. These approaches encourage relaxation, which may improve insulin sensitivity and help people better manage their diabetes-related stresses. Acupuncture is another alternative treatment that has shown promise in alleviating neuropathy symptoms and discomfort linked with diabetes complications.

Dietary therapies, such as low-carbohydrate or Mediterranean-style diets, have received attention for their beneficial impact on blood glucose levels and cardiovascular health. These techniques emphasize the significance of nutrient-dense meals, such as whole grains, fruits, vegetables, and healthy fats, which may help with glycemic management and general metabolic health.

Cinnamon and bitter melon have been studied for their possible hypoglycemic effects as herbal supplements. While research is continuing in this area, some studies indicate that some herbal medicines may help reduce blood glucose levels.

CHAPTER FIVE
Diabetes In Underserved Populations

Understanding and managing diabetes in vulnerable communities is critical for providing effective, culturally relevant treatment. Individuals with coexisting diseases, elderly folks, and people of different ethnic origins are examples of special populations.

Treatment approaches must be tailored to the specific requirements of these populations to maximize results and reduce health inequalities.

Diabetes management in older persons involves unique problems since aging is sometimes accompanied by other health concerns and drugs. When developing treatment regimens for this group, hypoglycemia, cognitive impairment, and functional restrictions must all be taken into account. Individualized techniques that take into consideration life expectancy, frailty, and general health are essential.

Addressing diabetes in varied ethnic groups requires an understanding of the role of genetics, lifestyle, and cultural variables in disease treatment. Individuals of African, Hispanic, or Asian heritage, for example, maybe more susceptible to certain diabetes-related problems. Education and treatment programs that are tailored to cultural preferences and dietary patterns might increase participation and adherence to prescribed actions.

Considerations For Children With Diabetes

Pediatric diabetes presents a unique combination of problems and concerns, necessitating specialized treatment to promote the well-being of diabetic children and adolescents. Diabetes care in this group necessitates a multidisciplinary approach that includes diet, mental health, and family dynamics in addition to medicine.

Involving parents or guardians in the treatment process and providing age-appropriate education are critical components of pediatric diabetes care. Healthcare practitioners must meet the particular emotional and developmental requirements of children and adolescents, creating a supportive atmosphere in which they may successfully manage their illnesses.

Continuous glucose monitoring (CGM) has shown to be an invaluable tool in the treatment of childhood diabetes, delivering real-time data to parents and healthcare practitioners. CGM enables timely insulin dose modifications, lowering the risk of hypoglycemia episodes and promoting tighter glycemic control.

This technology has altered diabetes care for children, making it more proactive and personalized.

Management Of Gestational Diabetes And Beyond

Gestational diabetes, which occurs during pregnancy, demands particular care to protect both mother and fetal health. To guarantee the best results for both mother and baby, effective gestational diabetes care includes a mix of lifestyle changes, blood glucose monitoring, and, in some situations, pharmaceutical therapies.

Nutritional counseling is important in gestational diabetes treatment because it helps pregnant women make appropriate food choices that help regulate blood glucose levels. Regular blood glucose monitoring, particularly after meals, allows for early modifications to dietary and lifestyle measures, reducing the risk of problems for both the mother and the growing baby.

When lifestyle changes are inadequate to maintain goal blood glucose levels, insulin treatment may be commenced. Close monitoring and coordination among obstetricians, endocrinologists, and diabetes educators are required to personalize treatment strategies to individual requirements while also addressing the possible influence of gestational diabetes on pregnancy and delivery outcomes.

Individuals with a history of gestational diabetes are at an elevated risk of getting type 2 diabetes later in life, even after the pregnancy has ended. Postpartum treatment and continuous lifestyle modifications are critical to reducing this risk, stressing the significance of long-term health for both mother and child.

Finally, the dynamic landscape of diabetes treatment continues to alter as new drugs, complementary therapies, and specialized methods for certain groups emerge. These improvements highlight the significance of a comprehensive and tailored approach to diabetes care, taking into account each individual's unique requirements and traits.

By remaining current on these advancements and adopting them into clinical practice, healthcare providers may help improve diabetes outcomes and quality of life.

CHAPTER SIX

Geriatric Diabetes: Personalized Care For Seniors

Diabetes is a chronic metabolic illness defined by increased blood sugar levels that affect people all over the globe. Diabetes in older persons, often known as geriatric diabetes, has increased significantly as the population ages.

This transformation has necessitated a critical rethinking of diabetes management, demanding specific ways to care for this fragile population.

Global Diabetes Management Perspectives

The growth of geriatric diabetes is not limited to one location; it is a worldwide problem. Various variables, such as changes in lifestyle, food habits, and greater life expectancy, all contribute to the global rise in diabetes among the elderly. With this global view, healthcare systems must adapt diabetes treatment techniques to varied cultural, socioeconomic, and healthcare infrastructure environments.

Various techniques are prioritized in different countries, including conventional medicine, community-based initiatives, and technology breakthroughs in diabetes treatment. Furthermore, identifying regional variations in access to healthcare and resources is critical in developing comprehensive geriatric diabetes treatment regimens.

Self-Management and Patient Empowerment

It is critical to empower older persons with diabetes via education and self-management measures. Encouraging patients to participate in their treatment improves results and quality of life. Empowerment includes educating patients about their disease, encouraging healthy lifestyle choices, and teaching self-monitoring and drug adherence skills.

Tailored support systems are critical for older persons, especially those with comorbidities or restricted mobility. Caregiver engagement, streamlined drug regimes, and assistive technology all play important roles in allowing efficient self-management in this population.

Diabetes Research And Treatment In The Future

Diabetes research and treatment are in a constant state of flux. Future diabetes care trends for older persons will focus on individualized therapy, leveraging technology breakthroughs, and researching novel therapeutics.

Tailoring therapy to an individual's genetic predispositions, comorbidities, and pharmaceutical response is a growing field of study. Furthermore, improvements in wearable technology and remote monitoring provide real-time health surveillance and intervention, enabling proactive diabetes control in older populations.

Novel therapy research, such as gene editing, regenerative medicine, and tailored drug delivery systems, offers the potential for more effective and less intrusive treatments. Furthermore, researchers are investigating the use of artificial intelligence and machine learning in anticipating diabetes complications and improving treatment approaches.

Conclusion

Finally, the paradigm of diabetes treatment for older persons demands a comprehensive approach. Global viewpoints emphasize the need for culturally sensitive, region-specific geriatric diabetes management practices. Patient empowerment via education and self-management continues to be critical in improving outcomes.

In the future, individualized approaches to diabetes management for older persons will rely on technology improvements and ongoing research into novel medications. Healthcare systems may successfully handle the problems presented by geriatric diabetes and enhance the well-being of older persons impacted by this illness by customizing care, stressing patient empowerment, and embracing future developments in research and treatment.